I0446252

KIDNEY DIALYSIS DIET COOKBOOK FOR BEGINNERS

The Complete Guide to Nourishing Low Sodium, Low Phosphorus and Low Potassium Kidney-friendly Recipes To Manage Renal Disease.

Joshua S. Gray

Copyright @ Joshua S. Gray 2023.

All rights reserved.
Before this document is duplicated or
reproduced in any manner. The publisher's
consent must be gained.
Therefore, the contents within can neither be
stored electronically, transferred, nor kept in a
database. Neither in part nor full can the
document be copied, scanned, faxed or retained
without approval from the publisher or creator.

For more information or help feel free to

contact me at:

joshuagrayhelpdesk@gmail.com

Table of Contents

TO GAIN ACCESS TO MORE BOOKS BY THE AUTHOR, SCAN THIS CODE.

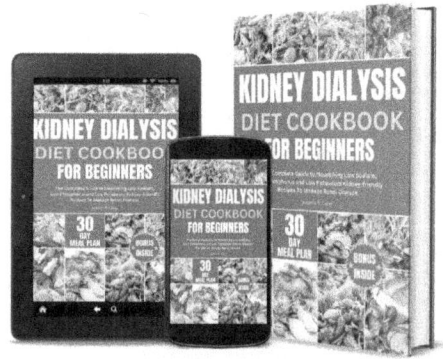

INTRODUCTION

Have you ever been in the kitchen and stared at an apparently never-ending list of dietary restrictions, wondering how you could make meals that would satisfy your cravings while still meeting your dialysis requirements? It's a challenge that many people encounter, and following a kidney dialysis diet can frequently feel like navigating a culinary maze.

Here's the really exciting part: what if I told you that the commonly held belief that flavor must be sacrificed for health when following this dietary path is untrue? What if mastering the technique of creating dishes that are delicious and customized to your specific health needs holds the key to managing your condition instead of bland food?

Welcome to the "Kidney Dialysis Diet Cookbook for Beginners," where you will discover delicious recipes to manage your condition. This cookbook aims to dispel the widespread belief that the only way to manage dialysis diets is to settle for boring, uninspired meals.

Imagine dining in a place where each bite is a flavorful celebration, where dietary restrictions open up new culinary possibilities, and where taking care of your health doesn't mean having to say goodbye to the pleasure of eating. What if I told you that you can actually access this flavorful and vibrant reality?

What if taking care of your kidneys was an exciting journey filled with trying out new flavors and textures instead of a difficult chore? What if the key to living well on a dialysis diet is to embrace the wealth of food options created just for you, rather than restricting yourself?

Within the pages of this cookbook, you will embark on an extraordinary journey. A guided tour through the flavors that make a kidney dialysis diet both manageable and enjoyable awaits you, along with a plethora of knowledge and expert insights and not just a collection of recipes.

I understand the challenges you face—the frustration, the confusion, and the desire for a resource that not only understands but also addresses the pains of managing a dialysis diet. This cookbook is crafted with you in mind, offering a compassionate approach to your culinary needs and providing practical solutions that extend beyond the kitchen.

Say goodbye to the misconception that flavor must be sacrificed in the pursuit of health. "Kidney Dialysis Diet Cookbook for Beginners" is not just a cookbook; it's your companion, your guide, and your ticket to a culinary experience that aligns with your health goals.

Get ready to go on a journey where every meal is an opportunity to take control of your health and enjoy the colorful tapestry of life. Your solution begins here.

CHAPTER 1

Understanding the Kidney Diet

Understanding the kidney diet is crucial for individuals with kidney-related conditions, such as chronic kidney disease (CKD) or those undergoing kidney dialysis. The primary goals of a kidney diet are to manage key nutrients like protein, phosphorus, potassium, sodium, and fluid intake to support kidney function and overall health. Here's a comprehensive overview:

1. Controlled Protein Intake:

- Why: Protein breakdown produces waste products that healthy kidneys eliminate. In compromised kidneys, excessive protein can strain their function.

- How: Limit high-protein foods, choose high-quality protein sources, and work with a dietitian to determine an individualized protein goal.

2. Phosphorus Management:

- Why: Impaired kidneys struggle to excrete excess phosphorus, leading to bone and heart issues.

- How: Limit high-phosphorus foods like dairy, nuts, seeds, and processed foods. Choose lower-phosphorus alternatives.

3. Potassium Regulation:

- Why: Too much potassium can disrupt heart rhythm. In kidney dysfunction, potassium levels may rise.

- How: Control potassium intake by limiting high-potassium foods like bananas, oranges, and potatoes. Portion control is crucial.

4. Sodium Restriction:

- Why: Sodium affects blood pressure and fluid balance. Kidney issues can lead to sodium retention.

- How: Minimize salt use, choose fresh foods over processed ones, and read labels for hidden sodium content.

5. Fluid Control:

- Why: Impaired kidneys may struggle to regulate fluid balance, leading to fluid retention or dehydration.

- How: Monitor fluid intake, including beverages and foods with high water content. Individualized recommendations are vital.

6. Balanced Carbohydrates:

- Why: Carbohydrates are a primary energy source. Focus on complex carbs, and limit refined sugars.

- How: Choose whole grains, fruits, and vegetables, and be mindful of added sugars.

7. Limiting Acidic Foods:

- Why: Kidneys play a role in maintaining acid-base balance. Limiting acidic foods can support this balance.

- How: Moderate intake of acidic foods like citrus fruits and tomatoes.

8. Individualized Nutrition:

- Why: Every person's nutritional needs are unique. Factors like age, weight, stage of kidney disease, and overall health impact dietary recommendations.

- How: Work closely with healthcare providers and dietitians for personalized advice and adjustments.

9. Cooking Techniques:

- Why: Certain cooking methods can enhance flavor without excessive use of salt or fats.

- How: Choose methods like grilling, roasting, and steaming. For more flavor, try experimenting with different herbs and spices.

10. Supervised Diet Management:

- Why: Kidney function can change over time. Regular monitoring and adjustments to the diet are essential.

- How: Attend regular check-ups, share concerns with healthcare providers, and adapt the diet as needed.

Understanding the kidney diet is an ongoing process that requires collaboration with healthcare professionals. This overview provides general insights, but individualized guidance is crucial for effective dietary management. Always consult with a healthcare provider or registered dietitian for personalized advice based on your specific health needs and circumstances.

The Role of Kidneys

The kidneys play a vital role in maintaining the overall health and homeostasis of the body. Here are some key functions and roles of the kidneys:

1. Filtration of Blood:

- Role: The primary function of the kidneys is to filter and remove waste products, toxins, and excess fluids from the blood to form urine.

- How: Blood is continuously circulated through the kidneys, and as it passes through nephrons (the functional units of the kidneys), waste products are filtered out.

2. Fluid and Electrolyte Balance:

- Role: The kidneys regulate the balance of water and electrolytes (such as sodium, potassium, and calcium) in the body.

- How: By adjusting the reabsorption and excretion of water and electrolytes, the kidneys help maintain proper fluid balance and electrolyte concentrations.

3. Acid-Base Balance:

- Role: The kidneys contribute to the regulation of the body's pH level by excreting hydrogen ions and reabsorbing bicarbonate ions.

- How: This process helps maintain the acid-base balance necessary for normal cellular function.

4. Blood Pressure Regulation:

- Role: The kidneys play a crucial role in regulating blood pressure by controlling the volume of blood and the amount of water excreted as urine.

- How: The renin-angiotensin-aldosterone system is activated to adjust blood pressure by influencing blood vessel constriction and fluid retention.

5. Erythropoiesis Regulation:

- Role: The kidneys produce and release erythropoietin, a hormone that stimulates the production of red blood cells in the bone marrow.

- How: Erythropoietin is released in response to low oxygen levels in the blood, helping maintain adequate oxygen-carrying capacity.

6. Metabolism of Vitamin D:

- Role: The kidneys convert inactive vitamin D into its active form, which is essential for the absorption of calcium and phosphate in the intestines.

- How: This process supports bone health and helps regulate calcium levels in the body.

7. Detoxification:

- Role: The kidneys filter and eliminate various metabolic byproducts, drugs, and toxins from the bloodstream.

- How: Through the filtration process, the kidneys remove substances that could be harmful if allowed to accumulate in the body.

8. Glucose Regulation:

- Role: The kidneys contribute to glucose homeostasis by reabsorbing glucose to prevent its loss in the urine.

- How: In situations of high blood glucose, the kidneys can reabsorb glucose to conserve it for energy.

9. Osmolality Regulation:

- Role: The kidneys adjust the concentration of urine to regulate osmolality, helping to conserve or eliminate water as needed.

- How: This process ensures that the body maintains proper hydration levels.

The kidneys play a critical role in maintaining the internal balance necessary for the proper functioning of the body. Dysfunction of the kidneys can lead to various health issues, emphasizing the importance of kidney health for overall well-being.

CHAPTER 2

Breakfast Recipes

1.   Mushroom and Red Pepper Omelet

Ingredients:

- 2 large eggs

- ¼ cup sliced mushrooms

- ¼ cup diced red pepper

- Salt and pepper to taste

Preparation:

1. Whisk eggs in a bowl and season with salt and pepper.

2. In a non-stick skillet, sauté mushrooms and red pepper until tender.

3. Pour whisked eggs over the vegetables and cook until set.

4. Fold the omelet in half and serve.

Nutritional Information:

(Per Serving)

- Calories: 180

- Protein: 15g

- Carbohydrates: 4g

- Fat: 12g

2.   Blueberry Muffins

Ingredients:

- 1 cup almond flour

- ¼ cup coconut flour

- ½ teaspoon baking soda

- ¼ teaspoon salt

- 3 large eggs

- ¼ cup coconut oil

- ¼ cup honey

- 1 teaspoon vanilla extract

- 1 cup fresh blueberries

Preparation:

1. Preheat oven to 350°F (175°C). Use paper liners to line a muffin tin.

2. In a bowl, mix almond flour, coconut flour, baking soda, and salt.

3. In a separate bowl, whisk eggs, then add coconut oil, honey, and vanilla extract.

4. Combine wet and dry ingredients, then fold in blueberries.

5. Divide batter into muffin cups and bake for 20-25 minutes.

Nutritional Information:

(Per Muffin)

- Calories: 180

- Protein: 5g

- Carbohydrates: 15g

- Fat: 12g

3. Chia Seed Pudding

Ingredients:

- 2 tablespoons chia seeds

- ½ cup almond milk

- ¼ teaspoon vanilla extract

- 1 teaspoon honey (optional)

- Fresh berries for topping

Preparation:

1. In a jar, mix chia seeds, almond milk, vanilla extract, and honey.

2. Stir well and let it cool in the fridge for at least 4 hours or overnight.

3. Top with fresh berries before serving.

Nutritional Information:

(Per Serving)

- Calories: 120

- Protein: 3g

- Carbohydrates: 12g

- Fat: 7g

4. Zucchini Bread

Ingredients:

- 2 cups grated zucchini
- ½ cup coconut flour
- ½ cup almond flour
- ½ teaspoon baking soda
- ¼ teaspoon salt
- 3 large eggs
- ¼ cup coconut oil
- ¼ cup honey
- 1 teaspoon cinnamon

Preparation:

1. Preheat oven to 350°F (175°C). Grease a loaf pan.

2. In a bowl, mix grated zucchini with a pinch of salt and let it sit for 10 minutes. Squeeze out excess moisture.

3. In another bowl, combine coconut flour, almond flour, baking soda, and cinnamon.

4. In a separate bowl, whisk eggs, then add coconut oil, honey, and squeezed zucchini.

5. Combine wet and dry ingredients, pour into the loaf pan, and bake for 45-50 minutes.

Nutritional Information:

(Per Slice)

- Calories: 160

- Protein: 5g

- Carbohydrates: 12g

- Fat: 10g

5. Lemon Berry Bread

- 1 cup almond flour

- ¼ cup coconut flour

- ½ teaspoon baking soda

- ¼ teaspoon salt

- 3 large eggs

- ¼ cup coconut oil

- ¼ cup honey

- Zest of 1 lemon

- 1 cup mixed berries

Preparation:

1. Preheat oven to 350°F (175°C). Grease a loaf pan.

2. In a bowl, mix almond flour, coconut flour, baking soda, and salt.

3. In a separate bowl, whisk eggs, then add coconut oil, honey, lemon zest, and mixed berries.

4. Combine wet and dry ingredients, pour into the loaf pan, and bake for 45-50 minutes.

Nutritional Information:

(Per Slice)

- Calories: 180

- Protein: 6g

- Carbohydrates: 14g

- Fat: 12g

6. Apple Bars

Ingredients:

- 2 cups grated apple
- ½ cup almond flour
- ½ cup coconut flour
- ½ teaspoon baking soda
- ¼ teaspoon salt
- 3 large eggs
- ¼ cup coconut oil
- ¼ cup honey
- 1 teaspoon cinnamon

Preparation:

1. Preheat oven to 350°F (175°C). Grease a baking dish.

2. In a bowl, mix grated apple with a pinch of salt and let it sit for 10 minutes. Squeeze out excess moisture.

3. In another bowl, combine almond flour, coconut flour, baking soda, and cinnamon.

4. In a separate bowl, whisk eggs, then add coconut oil, honey, and squeezed apple.

5. Combine wet and dry ingredients, pour into the baking dish, and bake for 30-35 minutes.

Nutritional Information:

(Per Bar)

- Calories: 150

- Protein: 4g

- Carbohydrates: 12g

- Fat: 9g

7. Breakfast Burrito

Ingredients:

- 2 large eggs, scrambled

- ¼ cup rinsed and drained black beans

- 2 tablespoons diced tomatoes

- 1 tablespoon diced onions

- 1 tablespoon chopped cilantro

- 1 whole-grain tortilla

Preparation:

1. In a skillet, scramble eggs until cooked.

2. Warm the tortilla in the skillet.

3. Assemble the burrito with scrambled eggs, black beans, tomatoes, onions, and cilantro.

4. Roll the burrito and serve.

Nutritional Information:

(Per Burrito)

- Calories: 280

- Protein: 15g

- Carbohydrates: 32g

- Fat: 12g

8. Cranberry Nut Bread

Ingredients:

- 1 cup almond flour
- ¼ cup coconut flour
- ½ teaspoon baking soda
- ¼ teaspoon salt
- 3 large eggs
- ¼ cup coconut oil
- ¼ cup honey
- 1 cup fresh or dried cranberries
- ½ cup of chopped nuts (e.g., pecans or walnuts)

Preparation:

1. Preheat oven to 350°F (175°C). Grease a loaf pan.

2. In a bowl, mix almond flour, coconut flour, baking soda, and salt.

3. In another bowl, whisk eggs, then add coconut oil, honey, cranberries, and chopped nuts.

4. Combine wet and dry ingredients, pour into the loaf pan, and bake for 45-50 minutes.

Nutritional Information:

(Per Slice)

- Calories: 190

- Protein: 6g

- Carbohydrates: 15g

- Fat: 12g

9. Peach Raspberry Smoothie

Ingredients:

- 1 cup frozen peaches
- ½ cup fresh or frozen raspberries
- ½ cup plain Greek yogurt
- ½ cup almond milk
- 1 tablespoon honey (optional)
- Ice cubes (optional)

Preparation:

1. Blend frozen peaches, raspberries, Greek yogurt, almond milk, and honey until smooth.
2. Add ice cubes if a colder consistency is desired.
3. Pour into a glass and enjoy.

Nutritional Information:

(Per Serving)

- Calories: 150

- Protein: 8g

- Carbohydrates: 22g

- Fat: 4g

10. Lemon Curd

Ingredients:

- 4 large eggs
- 1 cup fresh lemon juice
- Zest of 2 lemons
- ½ cup honey
- ½ cup coconut oil

Preparation:

1. In a heatproof bowl, whisk together eggs, lemon juice, lemon zest, and honey.

2. While the water simmers in the pot (double boiler), place the bowl over it and whisk constantly.

3. Gradually add coconut oil and continue whisking until the mixture thickens.

4. Remove from heat and let it cool before refrigerating.

Nutritional Information:

(Per Serving)

- Calories: 120

- Protein: 3g

- Carbohydrates: 10g

- Fat: 8g

CHAPTER 3

Seafood Recipes

1.   Baked Salmon with Herbed Quinoa Salad

Ingredients:

- 4 salmon fillets

- 1 cup quinoa, cooked

- Cherry tomatoes, halved

- Cucumber, diced

- Fresh herbs (such as parsley and dill)

- Lemon juice

- Olive oil

- Salt and pepper

Preparation:

1. Preheat oven to 375°F (190°C). Season salmon with salt and pepper and bake until cooked.

2. In a bowl, combine cooked quinoa, cherry tomatoes, cucumber, herbs, lemon juice, and olive oil.

3. Serve the baked salmon over the herbed quinoa salad.

Nutritional Information:

(Per Serving)

- Calories: 350

- Protein: 30g

- Carbohydrates: 25g

- Fat: 15g

2. Vegetable Fish Bake

Ingredients:

- White fish fillets

- Zucchini, sliced

- Cherry tomatoes, halved

- Red bell pepper, sliced

- Olive oil

- Garlic powder

- Lemon juice

- Fresh herbs like rosemary or thyme

- Salt and pepper

Preparation:

1. Preheat oven to 375°F (190°C). Place fish fillets in a baking dish.

2. Arrange sliced zucchini, cherry tomatoes, and red bell pepper around the fish.

3. Drizzle olive oil and lemon juice over the fish and vegetables. Sprinkle with fresh herbs, salt, garlic powder, and pepper.

4. Bake until the fish is cooked and the vegetables are tender.

Nutritional Information:

(Per Serving)

- Calories: 250

- Protein: 20g

- Carbohydrates: 10g

- Fat: 12g

3. Fish and Chips with Mushy Peas

Ingredients:

- White fish fillets

- Sweet potatoes, cut into fries

- Olive oil

- Paprika

- Frozen peas

- Mint leaves

- Lemon wedges

Preparation:

1. Preheat oven to 400°F (200°C). Toss sweet potato fries with olive oil and paprika, then bake until crispy.

2. Cook fish fillets according to preference.

3. For mushy peas, cook frozen peas and blend with mint leaves until smooth.

4. Serve fish and sweet potato fries with mushy peas and lemon wedges.

Nutritional Information:

(Per Serving)

- Calories: 300

- Protein: 25g

- Carbohydrates: 30g

- Fat: 10g

4. Seafood Corn Chowder

- Shrimp, peeled and deveined
- White fish, diced
- Corn kernels
- Potatoes, diced
- Onion, diced
- Garlic, minced
- Low-sodium vegetable broth
- Almond milk
- Fresh thyme
- Salt and pepper

Preparation:

1. In a pot, sauté onion and garlic. Add diced potatoes, corn, and vegetable broth. Simmer until potatoes are tender.

2. Add shrimp, diced fish, almond milk, fresh thyme, salt, and pepper. Simmer until seafood is cooked.

Nutritional Information:

(Per Serving)

- Calories: 220

- Protein: 18g

- Carbohydrates: 25g

- Fat: 7g

5. Baked Cod and Mushroom

Ingredients:

- Cod fillets

- Mushrooms, sliced

- Olive oil

- Garlic, minced

- Lemon juice

- Fresh parsley

- Salt and pepper

Preparation:

1. Preheat oven to 375°F (190°C). Place cod fillets in a baking dish.

2. In a skillet, sauté sliced mushrooms with olive oil and garlic. Spoon over the cod.

3. Drizzle lemon juice, sprinkle fresh parsley, salt, and pepper. Bake until the cod is cooked.

Nutritional Information:

(Per Serving)

- Calories: 180

- Protein: 22g

- Carbohydrates: 4g

- Fat: 8g

6. Eggplant Seafood Casserole

Ingredients:

- Eggplant, sliced
- Shrimp, peeled and deveined
- White fish, diced
- Tomato sauce (low-sodium)
- Garlic, minced
- Onion, diced
- Olive oil
- Fresh basil
- Salt and pepper

Preparation:

1. Preheat oven to 375°F (190°C). Sauté onion and garlic in olive oil. Add shrimp, diced fish, and cook until seafood is partially done.

2. In a baking dish, layer sliced eggplant, seafood mixture, and tomato sauce. Repeat layers.

3. Bake until eggplant is tender. Garnish with fresh basil, salt, and pepper.

Nutritional Information:

(Per Serving)

- Calories: 240

- Protein: 20g

- Carbohydrates: 15g

- Fat: 12g

7. Shrimp and Pasta Salad

Ingredients:

- Shrimp, cooked and peeled
- Whole-grain pasta, cooked
- Cherry tomatoes, halved
- Cucumber, diced
- Red onion, thinly sliced
- Olive oil
- Lemon juice
- Fresh dill
- Salt and pepper

Preparation:

1. In a bowl, combine cooked shrimp, pasta, cherry tomatoes, cucumber, and red onion.
2. Drizzle olive oil and lemon juice over the salad. Add fresh dill, salt, and pepper.

3. Toss the ingredients until well combined. Serve chilled.

Nutritional Information:

(Per Serving)

- Calories: 280

- Protein: 20g

- Carbohydrates: 35g

- Fat: 8g

8.   Seafood Gumbo

Ingredients:

- Shrimp, peeled and deveined
- Crab meat
- White fish, diced
- Okra, sliced
- Bell peppers, diced
- Celery, chopped
- Onion, diced
- Garlic, minced
- Low-sodium vegetable broth
- Cajun seasoning
- Brown rice

Preparation:

1. In a pot, sauté onion, garlic, bell peppers, and celery. Add okra, diced fish, crab meat, shrimp, and Cajun seasoning.

2. Pour in vegetable broth and simmer until seafood is cooked.

3. Serve over brown rice.

Nutritional Information:

(Per Serving)

- Calories: 320

- Protein: 25g

- Carbohydrates: 30g

- Fat: 10g

9. Codfish Burgers

- Cod fillets, cooked and flaked
- Whole-grain breadcrumbs
- Egg
- Dijon mustard
- Fresh parsley, chopped
- Olive oil
- Whole-grain buns
- Lettuce and tomato for topping

Preparation:

1. In a bowl, mix flaked cod, breadcrumbs, egg, Dijon mustard, and chopped parsley.

2. Form mixture into patties and cook in olive oil until golden brown.

3. Serve on whole-grain buns with lettuce and tomato.

Nutritional Information:

(Per Serving)

- Calories: 250

- Protein: 20g

- Carbohydrates: 25g

- Fat: 8g

10. Roasted Asparagus

Ingredients:

- Fresh asparagus spears

- Olive oil

- Garlic powder

- Lemon zest

- Salt and pepper

Preparation:

1. Preheat oven to 400°F (200°C). Toss asparagus spears with olive oil, garlic powder, lemon zest, salt, and pepper.

2. Roast in the oven until asparagus is tender and slightly crispy.

Nutritional Information:

(Per Serving)

- Calories: 50

- Protein: 3g

- Carbohydrates: 5g

- Fat: 3g

CHAPTER 4

Meat Recipes

1.   Ranch Chicken Pasta

Ingredients:

- Chicken breast, cooked and diced

- Whole-grain pasta

- Broccoli florets

- Cherry tomatoes, halved

- Greek yogurt-based ranch dressing

- Fresh dill

- Salt and pepper

Preparation:

1. Cook pasta according to package instructions. Drain and set aside.

2. In a bowl, combine cooked and diced chicken, pasta, broccoli, cherry tomatoes, and ranch dressing.

3. Garnish with fresh dill and season with salt and pepper.

Nutritional Information:

(Per Serving)

- Calories: 300

- Protein: 25g

- Carbohydrates: 35g

- Fat: 8g

2. Spicy Pork Chops with Apples

Ingredients:

- Pork chops
- Apples, sliced
- Olive oil
- Paprika
- Cinnamon
- Cayenne pepper
- Salt and pepper

Preparation:

1. Preheat oven to 375°F (190°C). Season pork chops with paprika, cinnamon, cayenne pepper, salt, and pepper.

2. In a skillet, sear pork chops in olive oil.

3. Transfer to a baking dish, top with sliced apples, and bake until pork is cooked.

Nutritional Information:

(Per Serving)

- Calories: 250

- Protein: 20g

- Carbohydrates: 15g

- Fat: 12g

3.   Chinese Chicken Salad

Ingredients:

- Chicken breast, cooked and shredded

- Napa cabbage, shredded

- Carrots, julienned

- Red bell pepper, thinly sliced

- Edamame

- Sesame seeds

- Low-sodium soy sauce

- Rice vinegar

- Sesame oil

- Fresh cilantro

Preparation:

1. In a large bowl, combine shredded chicken, Napa cabbage, carrots, bell pepper, and edamame.

2. In a small bowl, whisk together soy sauce, rice vinegar, and sesame oil. Pour over the salad.

3. Toss the salad, sprinkle with sesame seeds and fresh cilantro.

Nutritional Information:

(Per Serving)

- Calories: 280

- Protein: 25g

- Carbohydrates: 20g

- Fat: 10g

4.   Barley and Beef Stew

- Lean beef stew meat, cubed

- Barley, cooked

- Carrots, diced

- Celery, chopped

- Onion, diced

- Low-sodium beef broth

- Tomato paste

- Garlic, minced

- Fresh thyme

- Salt and pepper

Preparation:

1. In a pot, brown beef cubes. Add diced onions, garlic, carrots, and celery.

2. Stir in tomato paste, fresh thyme, salt, and pepper. Pour in beef broth.

3. Simmer until beef is tender. Add cooked barley before serving.

Nutritional Information:

(Per Serving)

- Calories: 300

- Protein: 28g

- Carbohydrates: 30g

- Fat: 8g

5.   Turkey Meatball Skewers

Ingredients:

- Ground turkey

- Whole-grain breadcrumbs

- Egg

- Fresh parsley, chopped

- Garlic powder

- Olive oil

- Cherry tomatoes

- Bell peppers, cut into chunks

Preparation:

1. In a bowl, mix ground turkey, breadcrumbs, egg, chopped parsley, and garlic powder.

2. Form mixture into meatballs and thread onto skewers with cherry tomatoes and bell peppers.

3. Grill or bake until meatballs are cooked through.

Nutritional Information:

(Per Serving)

- Calories: 220

- Protein: 20g

- Carbohydrates: 15g

- Fat: 10g

6.   Chicken and Rice Casserole

Ingredients:

- Chicken breast, cooked and shredded

- Brown rice, cooked

- Broccoli florets

- Low-fat cream of mushroom soup

- Low-sodium chicken broth

- Onion, diced

- Garlic, minced

- Olive oil

- Paprika

- Salt and pepper

Preparation:

1. Preheat oven to 350°F (175°C). In olive oil, sauté the onion and garlic until they are soft.

2. In a bowl, mix shredded chicken, cooked rice, broccoli, sautéed onions, and garlic.

3. In a separate bowl, mix cream of mushroom soup, chicken broth, paprika, salt, and pepper. Drizzle the chicken and rice mixture on top.

4. Transfer to a baking dish and bake until bubbly.

Nutritional Information:

(Per Serving)

- Calories: 280

- Protein: 25g

- Carbohydrates: 30g

- Fat: 8g

7. Turkey Waldorf Salad

Ingredients:

- Turkey breast, cooked and diced
- Apples, diced
- Celery, chopped
- Grapes, halved
- Walnuts, chopped
- Greek yogurt
- Lemon juice
- Honey

Preparation:

1. In a bowl, combine diced turkey, apples, celery, grapes, and chopped walnuts.

2. In a small bowl, mix Greek yogurt, lemon juice, and honey. Pour over the salad and toss.

Nutritional Information:

(Per Serving)

- Calories: 250

- Protein: 20g

- Carbohydrates: 25g

- Fat: 10g

8.   Spicy Frittata

- Eggs

- Egg whites

- Ground turkey

- Bell peppers, diced

- Onion, diced

- Spinach, chopped

- Hot sauce

- Olive oil

- Salt and pepper

Preparation:

1. Preheat oven to 375°F (190°C). In an oven-safe skillet, sauté diced onions, bell peppers, and ground turkey in olive oil.

2. Using a bowl, whisk the eggs and egg whites. Pour over the turkey and vegetable mixture.

3. Add chopped spinach and drizzle with hot sauce. Bake until the frittata is set.

Nutritional Information:

(Per Serving)

- Calories: 220

- Protein: 20g

- Carbohydrates: 10g

- Fat: 10g

9. Curried Turkey and Rice

Ingredients:

- Ground turkey
- Brown rice, cooked
- Onion, diced
- Garlic, minced
- Curry powder
- Coconut milk
- Frozen peas
- Fresh cilantro
- Olive oil
- Salt and pepper

Preparation:

1. In a skillet, sauté diced onions and garlic in olive oil. Add ground turkey and cook until browned.

2. Stir in curry powder, coconut milk, cooked brown rice, and frozen peas. Cook until heated through.

3. Garnish with fresh cilantro, salt, and pepper.

Nutritional Information:

(Per Serving)

- Calories: 280

- Protein: 22g

- Carbohydrates: 30g

- Fat: 10g

10. Honey Garlic Chicken

Ingredients:

- Chicken thighs, boneless and skinless
- Honey
- Soy sauce (low-sodium)
- Garlic, minced
- Ginger, grated
- Olive oil
- Green onions, sliced
- Sesame seeds

Preparation:

1. In a bowl, mix honey, soy sauce, minced garlic, and grated ginger. Marinate chicken thighs in the mixture.

2. In a skillet, heat olive oil and cook chicken until browned and cooked through.

3. Garnish with sliced green onions and sesame seeds before serving.

Nutritional Information:

(Per Serving)

- Calories: 250

- Protein: 22g

- Carbohydrates: 15g

- Fat: 12g

CHAPTER 5

Soup Recipes

1.   Thai Pumpkin Soup

Ingredients:

- Pumpkin, diced

- Coconut milk

- Vegetable broth (low-sodium)

- Ginger, grated

- Lemongrass, chopped

- Red curry paste

- Lime juice

- Fresh cilantro

- Salt and pepper

Preparation:

1. In a pot, combine diced pumpkin, coconut milk, vegetable broth, grated ginger, chopped lemongrass, and red curry paste.

2. Simmer until pumpkin is tender. Blend the soup until smooth.

3. Stir in lime juice, fresh cilantro, salt, and pepper.

Nutritional Information:

(Per Serving)

- Calories: 180

- Protein: 2g

- Carbohydrates: 20g

- Fat: 12g

2.   Carrot and Parsnip Soup

Ingredients:

- Carrots, diced

- Parsnips, diced

- Onion, diced

- Garlic, minced

- Low-sodium vegetable broth

- Fresh thyme

- Olive oil

- Salt and pepper

Preparation:

1. Sauté diced onions and garlic in olive oil. Add diced carrots and parsnips.

2. Pour in vegetable broth, add fresh thyme, and simmer until vegetables are tender.

3. Blend the soup until smooth. Season with salt and pepper.

Nutritional Information:

(Per Serving)

- Calories: 150

- Protein: 2g

- Carbohydrates: 25g

- Fat: 6g

3.　Curried Carrot Soup

- Carrots, sliced

- Onion, diced

- Garlic, minced

- Curry powder

- Low-sodium vegetable broth

- Coconut milk

- Fresh coriander

- Olive oil

- Salt and pepper

Preparation:

1. Sauté diced onions and garlic in olive oil. Add sliced carrots and curry powder.

2. Pour in vegetable broth and simmer until carrots are soft. Blend the soup until smooth.

3. Stir in coconut milk, fresh coriander, salt, and pepper.

Nutritional Information:

(Per Serving)

- Calories: 160

- Protein: 2g

- Carbohydrates: 20g

- Fat: 8g

4.   Chilled Cucumber Soup

Ingredients:

- Cucumbers, peeled and diced
- Greek yogurt
- Mint leaves
- Lemon juice
- Garlic, minced
- Low-sodium vegetable broth
- Olive oil
- Salt and pepper

Preparation:

1. In a blender, combine diced cucumbers, Greek yogurt, mint leaves, lemon juice, and minced garlic.

2. Blend until smooth. Add vegetable broth to achieve the desired consistency.

3. Chill the soup in the refrigerator. Before serving, drizzle with olive oil and add salt and pepper to taste.

Nutritional Information:

(Per Serving)

- Calories: 120

- Protein: 4g

- Carbohydrates: 15g

- Fat: 6g

5.   Vegetable and Lentil Soup

Ingredients:

- Lentils, rinsed

- Carrots, diced

- Celery, chopped

- Onion, diced

- Garlic, minced

- Low-sodium vegetable broth

- Tomatoes, diced

- Fresh thyme

- Olive oil

- Salt and pepper

Preparation:

1. Sauté diced onions and garlic in olive oil. Add carrots, celery, and lentils.

2. Pour in vegetable broth, add diced tomatoes and fresh thyme. Simmer until lentils are cooked.

3. Season with salt and pepper to make more appetising.

Nutritional Information:

(Per Serving)

- Calories: 200

- Protein: 10g

- Carbohydrates: 30g

- Fat: 4g

6.   Hearty Chicken Soup

Ingredients:

- Chicken breast, cooked and shredded

- Carrots, sliced

- Celery, chopped

- Onion, diced

- Garlic, minced

- Low-sodium chicken broth

- Brown rice, cooked

- Fresh parsley

- Olive oil

- Salt and pepper

Preparation:

1. Sauté diced onions and garlic in olive oil. Add sliced carrots, chopped celery, and shredded chicken.

2. Pour in chicken broth and simmer until vegetables are tender. Add cooked brown rice.

3. Garnish with fresh parsley, salt, and pepper.

Nutritional Information:

(Per Serving)

- Calories: 220

- Protein: 20g

- Carbohydrates: 25g

- Fat: 6g

7. Carrot and Sweet Potato Soup

Ingredients:

- Carrots, sliced

- Sweet potatoes, diced

- Onion, diced

- Garlic, minced

- Low-sodium vegetable broth

- Ginger, grated

- Coconut milk

- Fresh cilantro

- Olive oil

- Salt and pepper

Preparation:

1. Sauté diced onions and garlic in olive oil. Add sliced carrots and diced sweet potatoes.

2. Pour in vegetable broth, add grated ginger, and simmer until vegetables are soft.

3. Blend the soup until smooth. Stir in coconut milk, fresh cilantro, salt, and pepper.

Nutritional Information:

(Per Serving)

- Calories: 180

- Protein: 2g

- Carbohydrates: 25g

- Fat: 8g

8.   Borscht

- Beets, grated

- Cabbage, shredded

- Carrots, grated

- Onion, diced

- Garlic, minced

- Low-sodium vegetable broth

- Apple cider vinegar

- Fresh dill

- Olive oil

- Salt and pepper

Preparation:

1. Sauté diced onions and garlic in olive oil. Add grated beets, shredded cabbage, and grated carrots.

2. Pour in vegetable broth and simmer until vegetables are tender. Add apple cider vinegar.

3. Garnish with fresh dill, salt, and pepper.

Nutritional Information:

(Per Serving)

- Calories: 160

- Protein: 3g

- Carbohydrates: 25g

- Fat: 6g

9. Vegetable Laksa Soup

- Rice noodles

- Coconut milk

- Vegetable broth (low-sodium)

- Red curry paste

- Tofu, cubed

- Bean sprouts

- Bok choy, chopped

- Lime wedges

- Fresh cilantro

- Olive oil

- Salt and pepper

Preparation:

1. Cook rice noodles according to package instructions. Set aside.

2. In a pot, combine coconut milk, vegetable broth, red curry paste, and cubed tofu. Simmer until tofu is cooked.

3. Add cooked rice noodles, bean sprouts, and chopped bok choy. Serve with lime wedges and garnish with fresh cilantro.

Nutritional Information:

(Per Serving)

- Calories: 250

- Protein: 10g

- Carbohydrates: 30g

- Fat: 10g

10. Pear and Cauliflower Soup

Ingredients:

- Pears, peeled and diced

- Cauliflower, chopped

- Onion, diced

- Garlic, minced

- Low-sodium vegetable broth

- Almond milk

- Curry powder

- Nutmeg

- Olive oil

- Salt and pepper

Preparation:

1. Sauté diced onions and garlic in olive oil. Add chopped cauliflower and diced pears.

2. Pour in vegetable broth and simmer until vegetables are soft. Blend the soup until smooth.

3. Stir in almond milk, curry powder, nutmeg, salt, and pepper.

Nutritional Information:

(Per Serving)

- Calories: 150

- Protein: 2g

- Carbohydrates: 30g

- Fat: 4g

CHAPTER 6

Dessert Recipes

1. Apple and Blueberry Crisp

Ingredients:

- Apples, peeled and sliced
- Blueberries
- Whole oats
- Almond flour
- Coconut oil
- Cinnamon
- Nutmeg
- Maple syrup

Preparation:

1. In a bowl, combine sliced apples and blueberries. Place in a baking dish.

2. In a separate bowl, mix whole oats, almond flour, melted coconut oil, cinnamon, nutmeg, and maple syrup.

3. Spread the oat mixture over the fruit. Bake until the top is golden and fruit is bubbly.

Nutritional Information:

(Per Serving)

- Calories: 180

- Protein: 3g

- Carbohydrates: 30g

- Fat: 7g

2. Raspberry Pear Sorbet

Ingredients:

- Raspberries

- Pears, peeled and diced

- Lemon juice

- Agave syrup

Preparation:

1. Blend raspberries, diced pears, lemon juice, and agave syrup until smooth.

2. Freeze the mixture after pouring it into a shallow dish. Stir every 30 minutes until set.

Nutritional Information:

(Per Serving)

- Calories: 120

- Protein: 1g

- Carbohydrates: 30g

- Fat: 0.5g

3.   Strawberry Rugelach

Ingredients:

- Whole-wheat flour

- Cream cheese

- Butter

- Strawberries, sliced

- Cinnamon

- Honey

Preparation:

1. Mix whole-wheat flour, cream cheese, and butter to form a dough. Roll out into a circle.

2. Spread sliced strawberries over the dough. Drizzle with honey and sprinkle with cinnamon.

3. Cut into wedges and roll each wedge. Bake until golden.

Nutritional Information:

(Per Serving)

- Calories: 150

- Protein: 2g

- Carbohydrates: 20g

- Fat: 8g

4.   Spicy Peaches

Ingredients:

- Peaches, sliced

- Cinnamon

- Nutmeg

- Honey

- Greek yogurt

Preparation:

1. In a bowl, mix sliced peaches, cinnamon, nutmeg, and honey.

2. Sauté the peach mixture until softened. Serve with a dollop of Greek yogurt.

Nutritional Information:

(Per Serving)

- Calories: 100

- Protein: 3g

- Carbohydrates: 25g

- Fat: 1g

5.   Apple Cinnamon Chips

- Apples, thinly sliced

- Cinnamon

- Stevia

Preparation:

1. Preheat oven to 200°F (95°C). On a baking sheet, arrange the apple slices.

2. Sprinkle with cinnamon and stevia. Bake until crispy.

Nutritional Information:

(Per Serving)

- Calories: 50

- Protein: 0.5g

- Carbohydrates: 15g

- Fat: 0.5g

6.   Strawberry Sorbet

Ingredients:

- Strawberries

- Lemon juice

- Agave syrup

Preparation:

1. Blend strawberries, lemon juice, and agave syrup until smooth.

2. Freeze the mixture after pouring it into a shallow dish. Stir every 30 minutes until set.

Nutritional Information:

(Per Serving)

- Calories: 80

- Protein: 1g

- Carbohydrates: 20g

- Fat: 0.5g

7.   Apple Fritter Rings

Ingredients:

- Apples, cored and sliced

- Whole-wheat flour

- Cinnamon

- Nutmeg

- Almond milk

- Maple syrup

Preparation:

1. In a bowl, mix whole-wheat flour, cinnamon, nutmeg, almond milk, and maple syrup.

2. Dip apple slices into the batter and fry until golden.

Nutritional Information:

(Per Serving)

- Calories: 120

- Protein: 1g

- Carbohydrates: 25g

- Fat: 2g

8. Sweet Cherry Cobbler

- Sweet cherries, pitted

- Whole-wheat flour

- Baking powder

- Almond milk

- Maple syrup

- Vanilla extract

Preparation:

1. In a baking dish, arrange pitted sweet cherries.

2. In a bowl, mix whole-wheat flour, baking powder, almond milk, maple syrup, and vanilla extract. Pour over the cherries.

3. Bake until the top is golden and cherries are bubbly.

Nutritional Information:

(Per Serving)

- Calories: 150

- Protein: 2g

- Carbohydrates: 30g

- Fat: 2.5g

9. Poached Pears

Ingredients:

- Pears, peeled and halved

- Red wine

- Cinnamon

- Star anise

- Honey

- Greek yogurt

Preparation:

1. In a pot, combine red wine, cinnamon, star anise, and honey. Bring to a simmer.

2. Add peeled and halved pears. Poach until tender. Serve with a dollop of Greek yogurt.

Nutritional Information:

(Per Serving)

- Calories: 120

- Protein: 2g

- Carbohydrates: 25g

- Fat: 0.5g

10. Warm Bread Pudding

Ingredients:

- Whole-wheat bread, cubed

- Almond milk

- Eggs

- Vanilla extract

- Cinnamon

- Raisins

- Maple syrup

Preparation:

1. In a bowl, whisk together almond milk, eggs, vanilla extract, and cinnamon.

2. Add cubed whole-wheat bread and raisins. Let it soak.

3. Transfer to a baking dish, drizzle with maple syrup, and bake until set.

Nutritional Information:

(Per Serving)

- Calories: 180

- Protein: 5g

- Carbohydrates: 30g

- Fat: 4g

30 Day Meal Plan

Week 1

Day 1:

Breakfast: Blueberry Muffins

Lunch: Baked Salmon with Herbed Quinoa Salad

Dinner: Ranch Chicken Pasta

Soup: Thai Pumpkin Soup

Dessert: Apple and Blueberry Crisp

Day 2:

Breakfast: Chia Seed Pudding

Lunch: Tuna and Olive Tapenade Wrap

Dinner: Spicy Pork Chops with Apples

Soup: Carrot and Parsnip Soup

Dessert: Raspberry Pear Sorbet

Day 3:

Breakfast: Zucchini Bread

Lunch: Vegetable Fish Bake

Dinner: Chinese Chicken Salad

Soup: Curried Carrot Soup

Dessert: Strawberry Rugelach

Day 4:

Breakfast: Lemon Berry Bread

Lunch: Fish and Chips with Mushy Peas

Dinner: Barley and Beef Stew

Soup: Chilled Cucumber Soup

Dessert: Spicy Peaches

Day 5:

Breakfast: Apple Bars

Lunch: Eggplant Seafood Casserole

Dinner: Turkey Meatball Skewers

Soup: Vegetable and Lentil Soup

Dessert: Apple Cinnamon Chips

Day 6:

Breakfast: Breakfast Burrito

Lunch: Shrimp and Pasta Salad

Dinner: Chicken and Rice Casserole

Soup: Hearty Chicken Soup

Dessert: Strawberry Sorbet

Day 7:

Breakfast: Cranberry Nut Bread

Lunch: Seafood Gumbo

Dinner: Turkey Waldorf Salad

Soup: Carrot and Sweet Potato Soup

Dessert: Apple Fritter Rings

Week 2

Breakfast: Zucchini Bread

Lunch: Vegetable Fish Bake

Dinner: Chinese Chicken Salad

Soup: Curried Carrot Soup

Dessert: Strawberry Rugelach

Breakfast: Lemon Berry Bread

Lunch: Fish and Chips with Mushy Peas

Dinner: Barley and Beef Stew

Soup: Chilled Cucumber Soup

Dessert: Spicy Peaches

Day 10:

Breakfast: Blueberry Muffins

Lunch: Baked Salmon with Herbed Quinoa Salad

Dinner: Ranch Chicken Pasta

Soup: Thai Pumpkin Soup

Dessert: Apple and Blueberry Crisp

Day 11:

Breakfast: Chia Seed Pudding

Lunch: Tuna and Olive Tapenade Wrap

Dinner: Spicy Pork Chops with Apples

Soup: Carrot and Parsnip Soup

Dessert: Raspberry Pear Sorbet

Day 12:

Breakfast: Cranberry Nut Bread

Lunch: Seafood Gumbo

Dinner: Turkey Waldorf Salad

Soup: Carrot and Sweet Potato Soup

Dessert: Apple Fritter Rings

Day 13:

Breakfast: Blueberry Muffins

Lunch: Baked Salmon with Herbed Quinoa Salad

Dinner: Ranch Chicken Pasta

Soup: Thai Pumpkin Soup

Dessert: Apple and Blueberry Crisp

Day 14:

Breakfast: Chia Seed Pudding

Lunch: Tuna and Olive Tapenade Wrap

Dinner: Spicy Pork Chops with Apples

Soup: Carrot and Parsnip Soup

Dessert: Raspberry Pear Sorbet

Week 3

Breakfast: Zucchini Bread

Lunch: Vegetable Fish Bake

Dinner: Chinese Chicken Salad

Soup: Curried Carrot Soup

Dessert: Strawberry Rugelach

Breakfast: Lemon Berry Bread

Lunch: Fish and Chips with Mushy Peas

Dinner: Barley and Beef Stew

Soup: Chilled Cucumber Soup

Dessert: Spicy Peaches

Day 17:

Breakfast: Apple Bars

Lunch: Eggplant Seafood Casserole

Dinner: Turkey Meatball Skewers

Soup: Vegetable and Lentil Soup

Dessert: Apple Cinnamon Chips

Day 18:

Breakfast: Breakfast Burrito

Lunch: Shrimp and Pasta Salad

Dinner: Chicken and Rice Casserole

Soup: Hearty Chicken Soup

Dessert: Strawberry Sorbet

Day 19:

Breakfast: Cranberry Nut Bread

Lunch: Seafood Gumbo

Dinner: Turkey Waldorf Salad

Soup: Carrot and Sweet Potato Soup

Dessert: Apple Fritter Rings

Day 20:

Breakfast: Lemon Berry Bread

Lunch: Fish and Chips with Mushy Peas

Dinner: Barley and Beef Stew

Soup: Chilled Cucumber Soup

Dessert: Spicy Peaches

Day 21:

Breakfast: Apple Bars

Lunch: Eggplant Seafood Casserole

Dinner: Turkey Meatball Skewers

Soup: Vegetable and Lentil Soup

Dessert: Apple Cinnamon Chips

Week 4

Breakfast: Blueberry Muffins

Lunch: Baked Salmon with Herbed Quinoa Salad

Dinner: Ranch Chicken Pasta

Soup: Thai Pumpkin Soup

Dessert: Apple and Blueberry Crisp

Breakfast: Chia Seed Pudding

Lunch: Tuna and Olive Tapenade Wrap

Dinner: Spicy Pork Chops with Apples

Soup: Carrot and Parsnip Soup

Dessert: Raspberry Pear Sorbet

Day 24:

Breakfast: Zucchini Bread

Lunch: Vegetable Fish Bake

Dinner: Chinese Chicken Salad

Soup: Curried Carrot Soup

Dessert: Strawberry Rugelach

Day 25:

Breakfast: Lemon Berry Bread

Lunch: Fish and Chips with Mushy Peas

Dinner: Barley and Beef Stew

Soup: Chilled Cucumber Soup

Dessert: Spicy Peaches

Day 26:

Breakfast: Apple Bars

Lunch: Eggplant Seafood Casserole

Dinner: Turkey Meatball Skewers

Soup: Vegetable and Lentil Soup

Dessert: Apple Cinnamon Chips

Day 27:

Breakfast: Breakfast Burrito

Lunch: Shrimp and Pasta Salad

Dinner: Chicken and Rice Casserole

Soup: Hearty Chicken Soup

Dessert: Strawberry Sorbet

Day 28:

Breakfast: Cranberry Nut Bread

Lunch: Seafood Gumbo

Dinner: Turkey Waldorf Salad

Soup: Carrot and Sweet Potato Soup

Dessert: Apple Fritter Rings

Day 29:

Breakfast: Zucchini Bread

Lunch: Vegetable Fish Bake

Dinner: Chinese Chicken Salad

Soup: Curried Carrot Soup

Dessert: Strawberry Rugelach

Day 30:

Breakfast: Breakfast Burrito

Lunch: Shrimp and Pasta Salad

Dinner: Chicken and Rice Casserole

Soup: Hearty Chicken Soup

Dessert: Strawberry Sorbet

CONCLUSION

As we approach the last pages of this cookbook, I would like to sincerely thank you for starting this path to a happier, healthier life. It is very admirable that you are dedicated to finding recipes that are kidney-friendly and changing your diet for the better.

Handling the difficulties associated with kidney health calls for commitment and a careful consideration of our diet. It is my sincere wish that the recipes in this cookbook have not only whetted your appetite but also opened your eyes to a newfound sense of wellbeing.

You have a manual that can help you live a healthier lifestyle in your hands, not just a cookbook. I hope that each dish in these pages, as you explore the variety of flavors and healthy ingredients, not only satisfies your hunger but also makes you feel happy and content.

Never forget that decisions you make today have a big impact on tomorrow. Your health is a valuable asset. This cookbook will prove to be an invaluable tool in helping you overcome any obstacles you may encounter along the way to optimal kidney health.

Wishing you wellness, fulfillment, and many delicious moments as you continue on this path. Thank you for entrusting me with a role in your pursuit of a healthier life.

My Little Request

Dear Reader,

Thanks for your purchase, I hope you enjoyed reading.

Could you please take a few seconds to leave a positive feedback on this book?

It'll help reach more people and we can collectively help reverse this deadly disease.

Thank you.

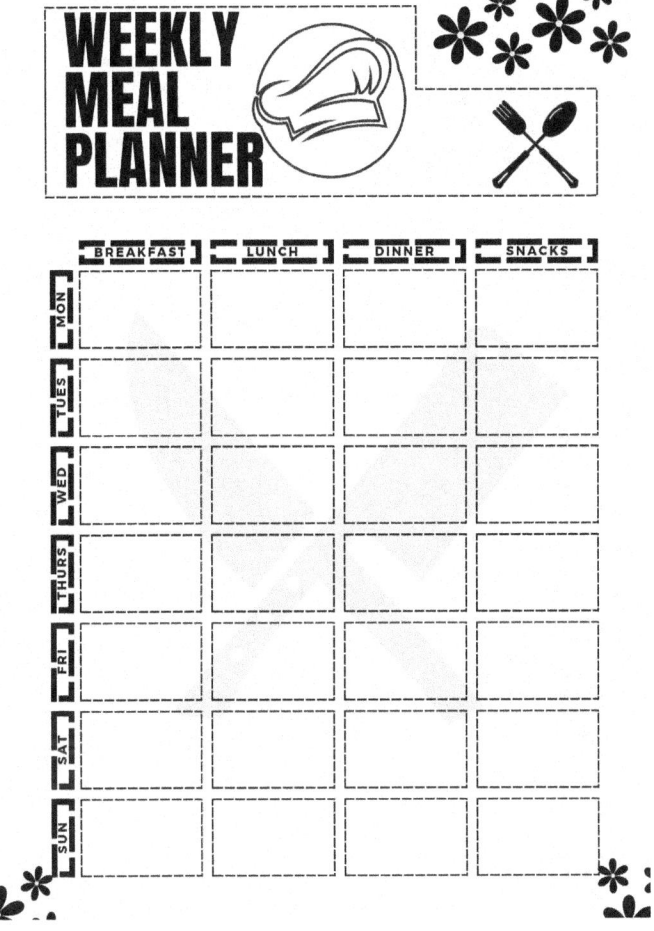

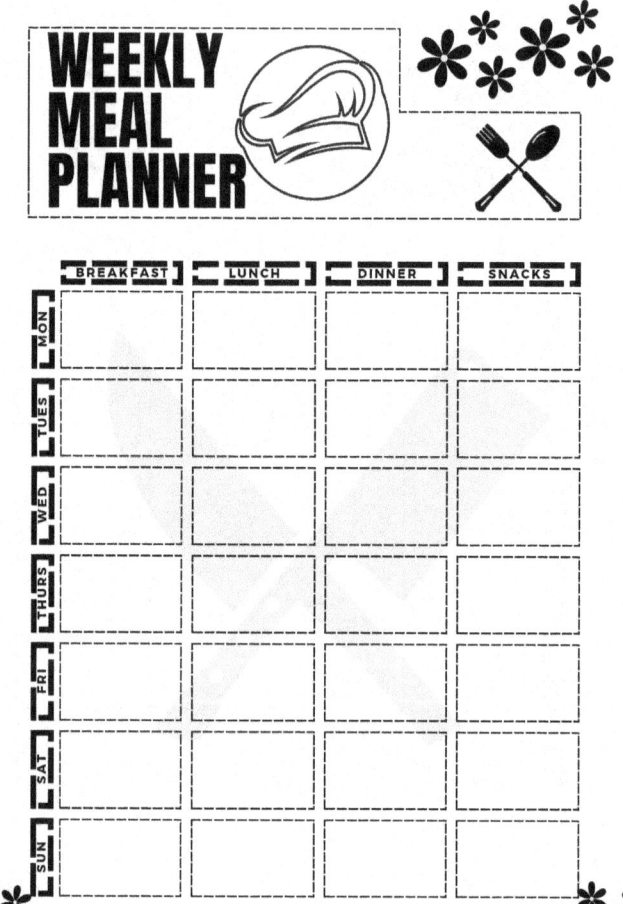

WEEKLY MEAL PLANNER

	BREAKFAST	LUNCH	DINNER	SNACKS
MON				
TUES				
WED				
THURS				
FRI				
SAT				
SUN				

KIDNEY DIALYSIS DIET COOKBOOK FOR BEGINNERS

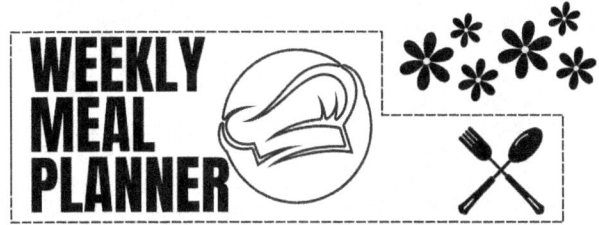

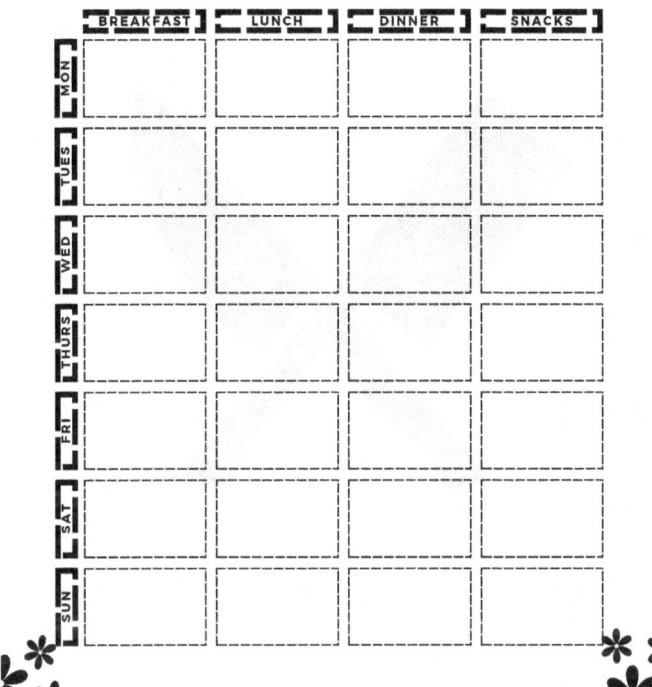

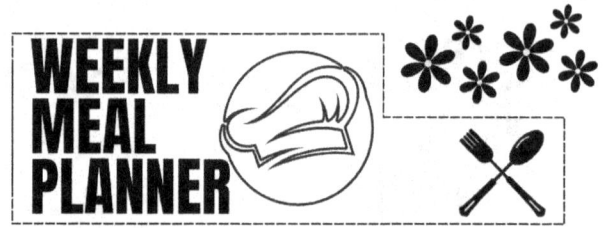

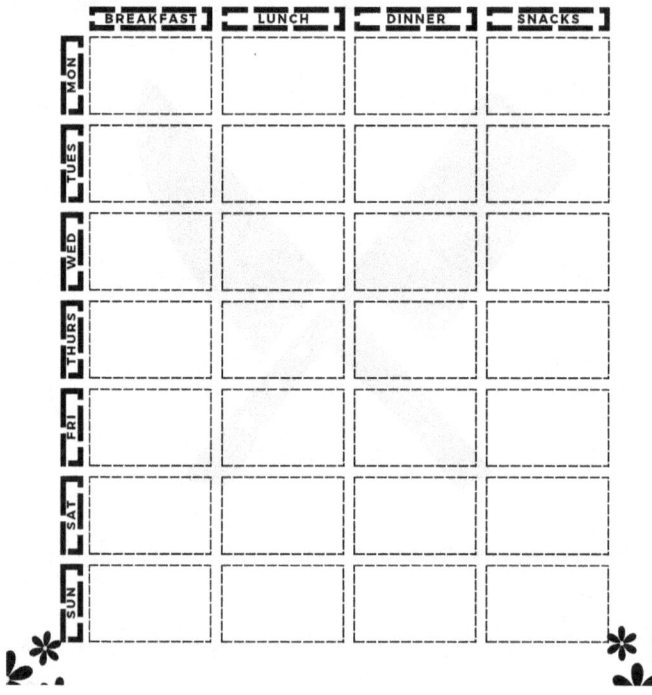

	BREAKFAST	LUNCH	DINNER	SNACKS
MON				
TUES				
WED				
THURS				
FRI				
SAT				
SUN				

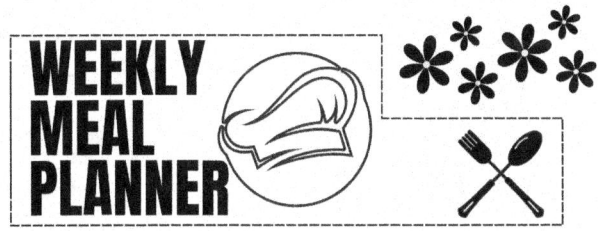

WEEKLY MEAL PLANNER

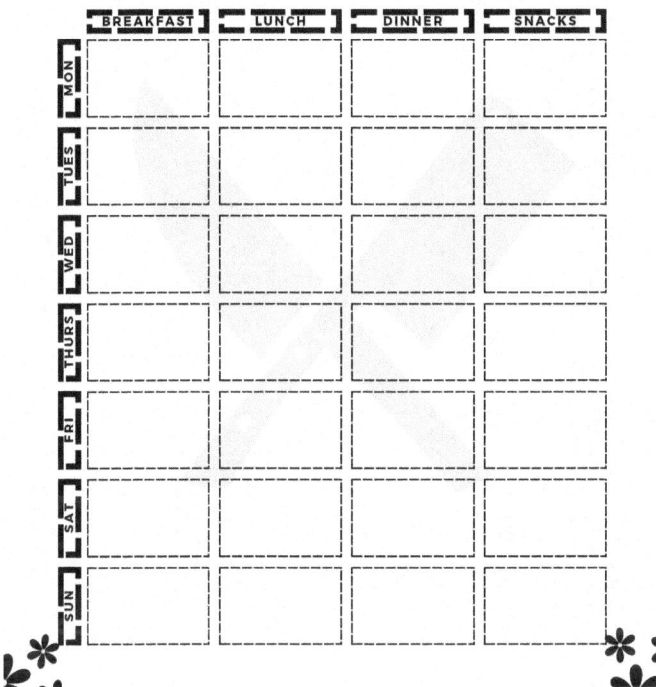

	BREAKFAST	LUNCH	DINNER	SNACKS
MON				
TUES				
WED				
THURS				
FRI				
SAT				
SUN				

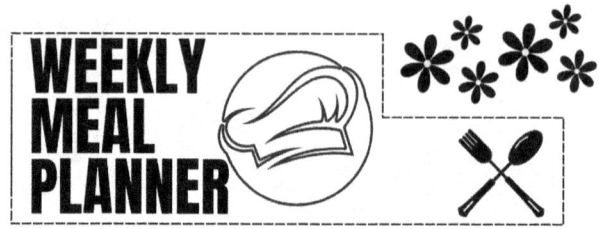

	BREAKFAST	LUNCH	DINNER	SNACKS
MON				
TUES				
WED				
THURS				
FRI				
SAT				
SUN				

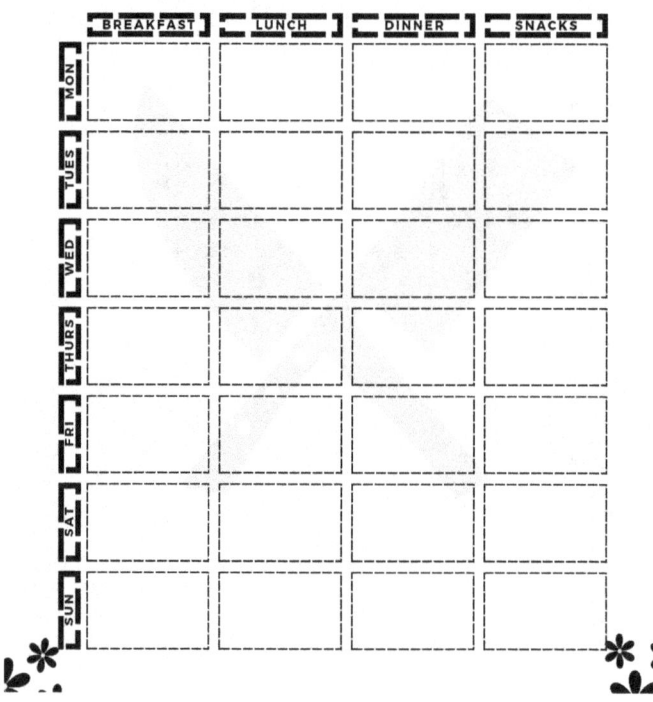

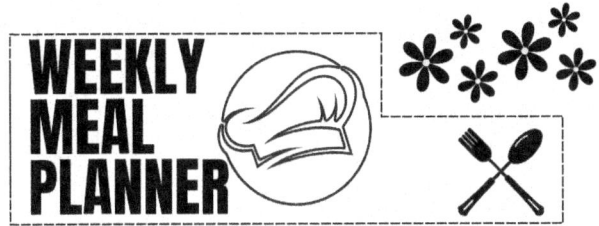

WEEKLY MEAL PLANNER

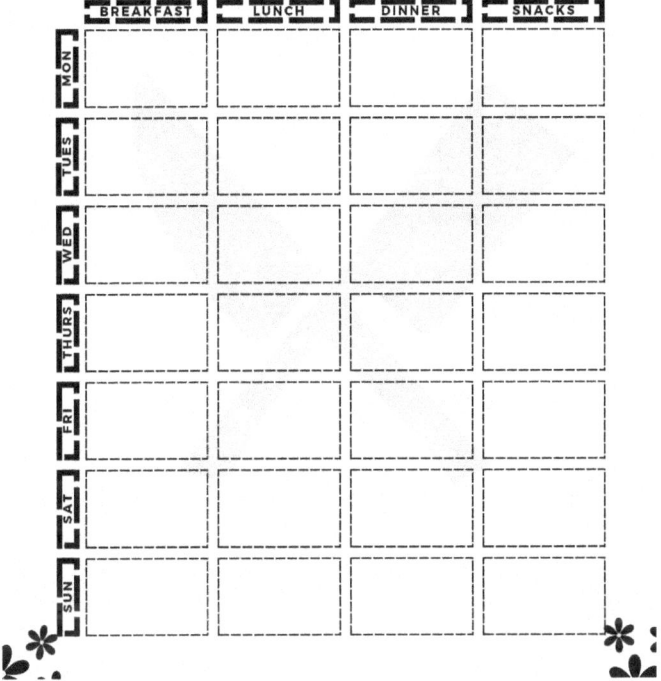

	BREAKFAST	LUNCH	DINNER	SNACKS
MON				
TUES				
WED				
THURS				
FRI				
SAT				
SUN				

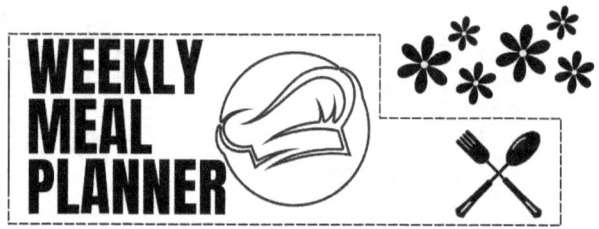

WEEKLY MEAL PLANNER

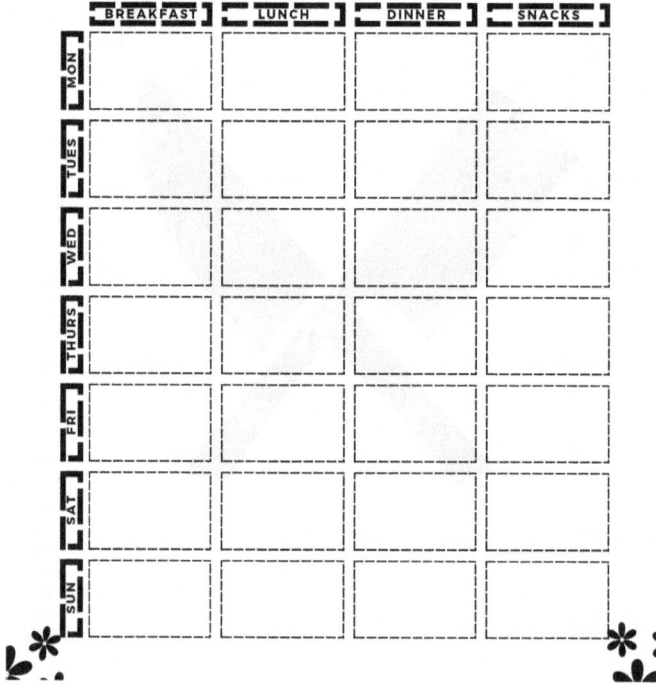

	BREAKFAST	LUNCH	DINNER	SNACKS
MON				
TUES				
WED				
THURS				
FRI				
SAT				
SUN				

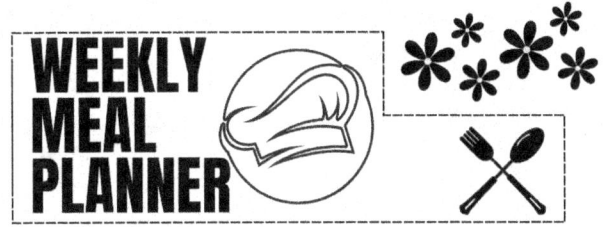

	BREAKFAST	LUNCH	DINNER	SNACKS
MON				
TUES				
WED				
THURS				
FRI				
SAT				
SUN				

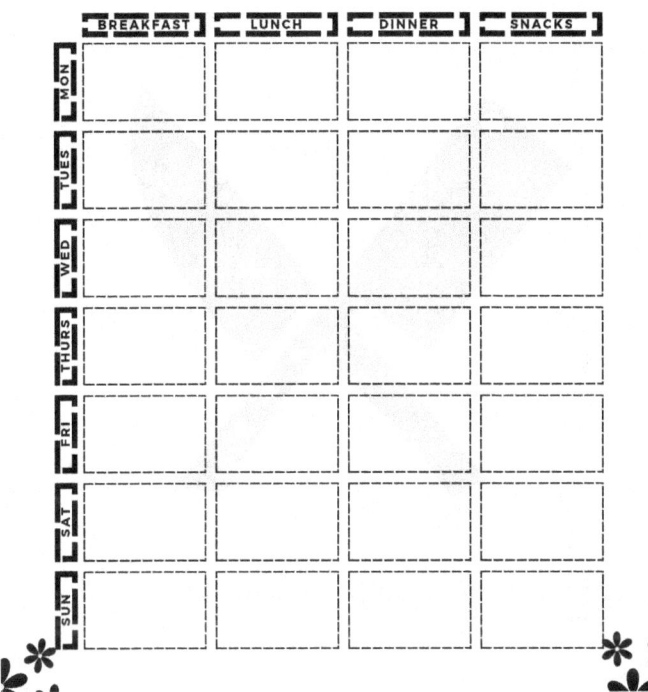

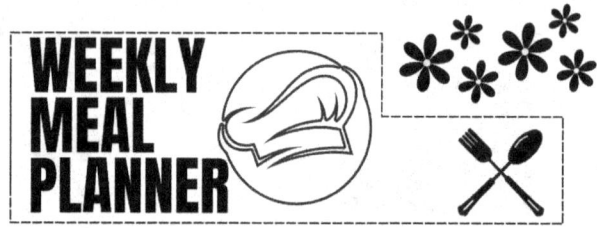

WEEKLY MEAL PLANNER

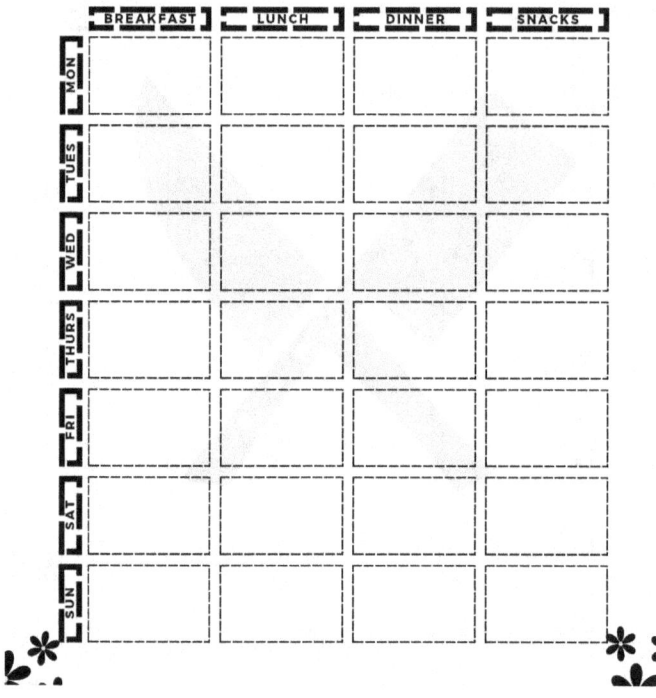

	BREAKFAST	LUNCH	DINNER	SNACKS
MON				
TUES				
WED				
THURS				
FRI				
SAT				
SUN				

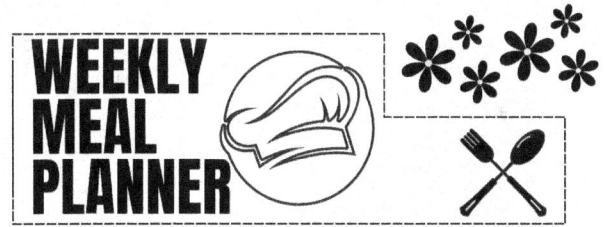

WEEKLY MEAL PLANNER

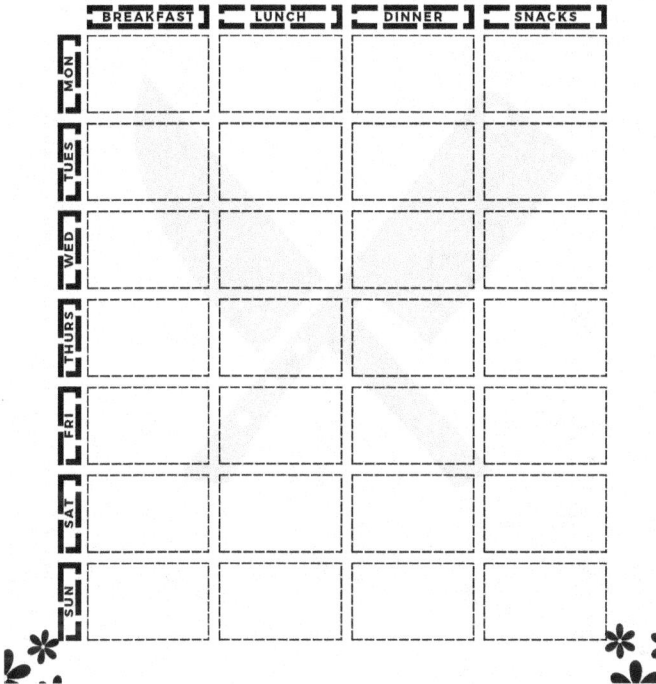

	BREAKFAST	LUNCH	DINNER	SNACKS
MON				
TUES				
WED				
THURS				
FRI				
SAT				
SUN				

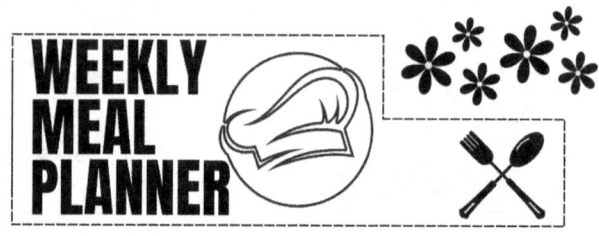

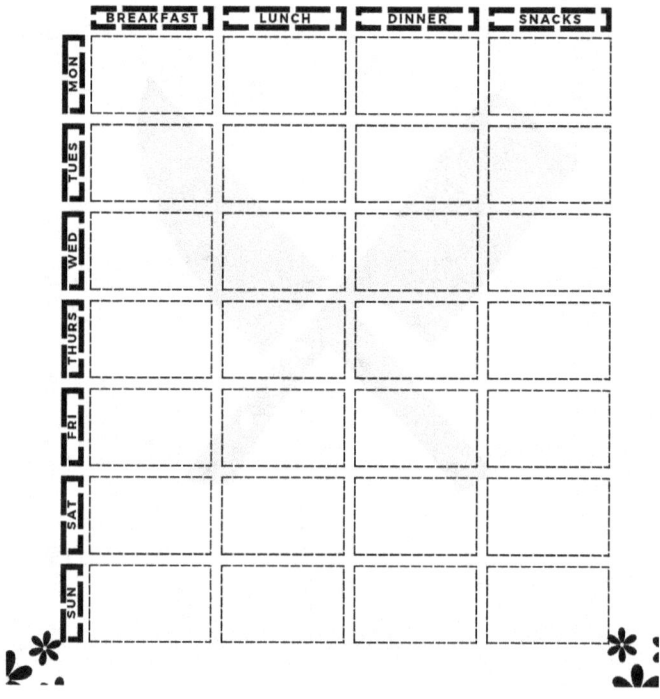

	BREAKFAST	LUNCH	DINNER	SNACKS
MON				
TUES				
WED				
THURS				
FRI				
SAT				
SUN				

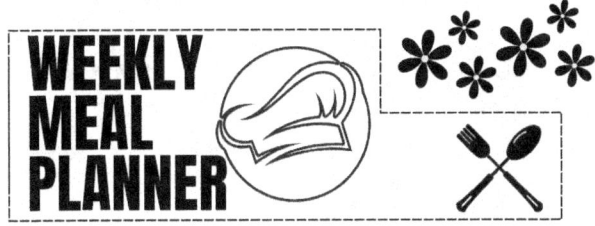

WEEKLY MEAL PLANNER

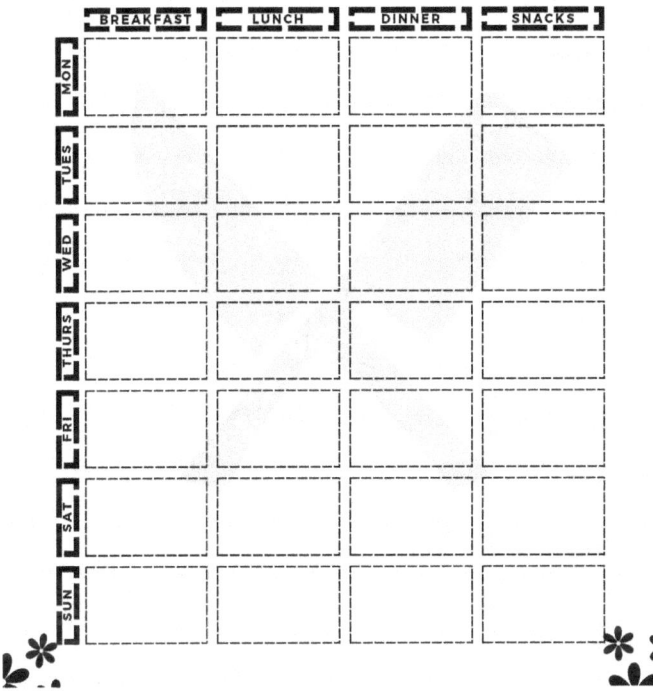

	BREAKFAST	LUNCH	DINNER	SNACKS
MON				
TUES				
WED				
THURS				
FRI				
SAT				
SUN				

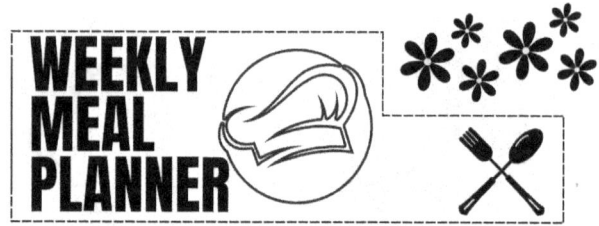

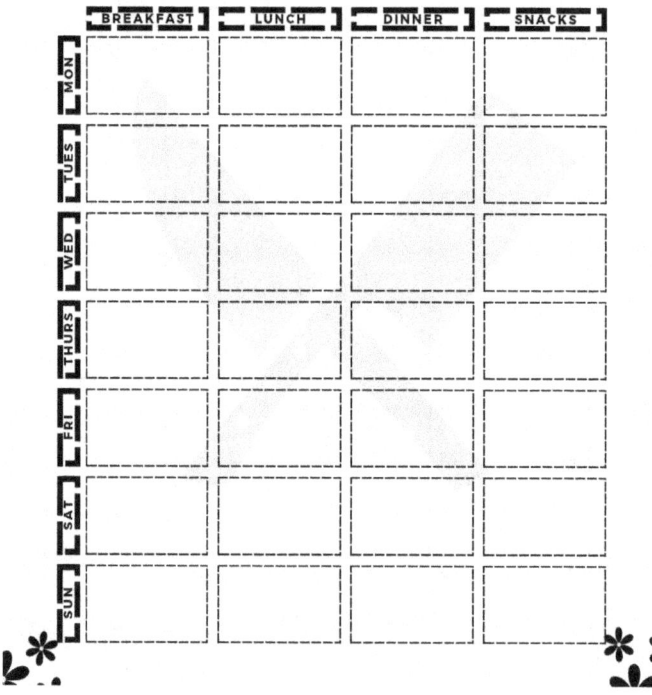

	BREAKFAST	LUNCH	DINNER	SNACKS
MON				
TUES				
WED				
THURS				
FRI				
SAT				
SUN				

KIDNEY DIALYSIS DIET COOKBOOK FOR BEGINNERS

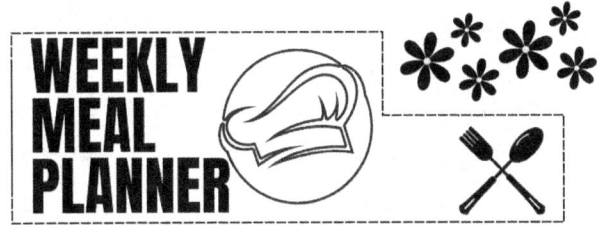

WEEKLY MEAL PLANNER

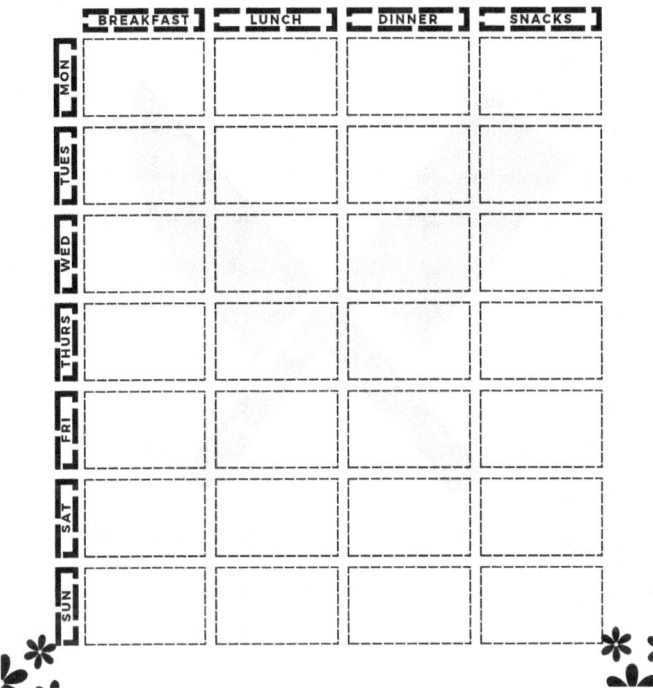

	BREAKFAST	LUNCH	DINNER	SNACKS
MON				
TUES				
WED				
THURS				
FRI				
SAT				
SUN				

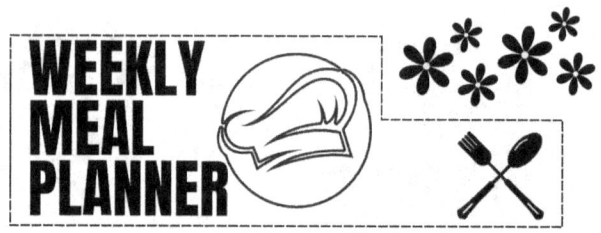

WEEKLY MEAL PLANNER

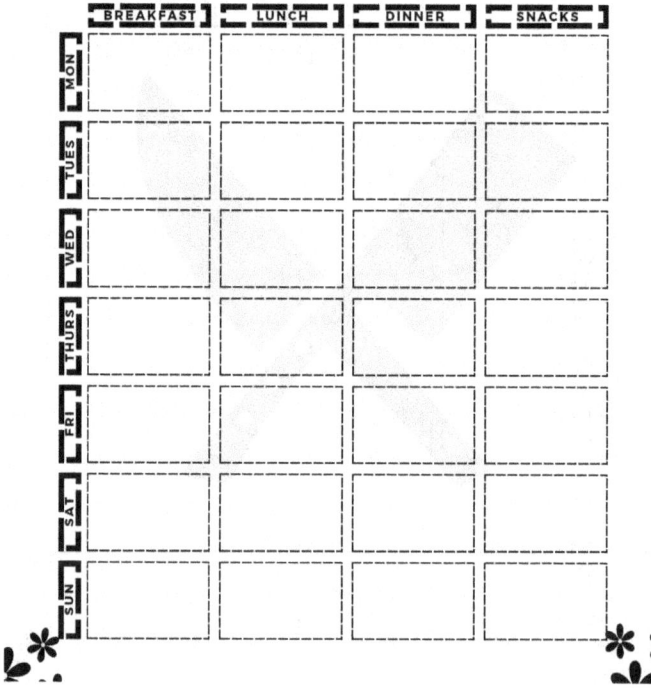

	BREAKFAST	LUNCH	DINNER	SNACKS
MON				
TUES				
WED				
THURS				
FRI				
SAT				
SUN				

KIDNEY DIALYSIS DIET COOKBOOK FOR BEGINNERS

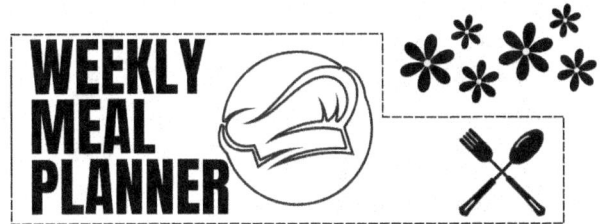

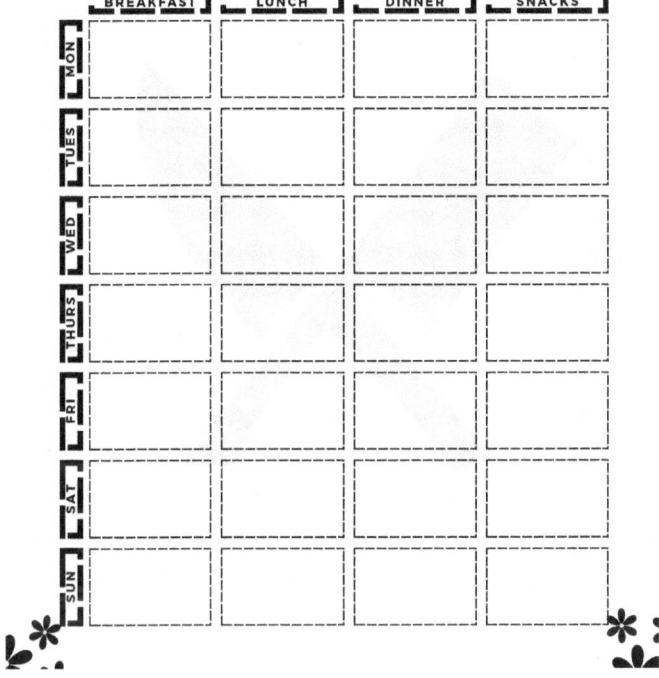

	BREAKFAST	LUNCH	DINNER	SNACKS
MON				
TUES				
WED				
THURS				
FRI				
SAT				
SUN				

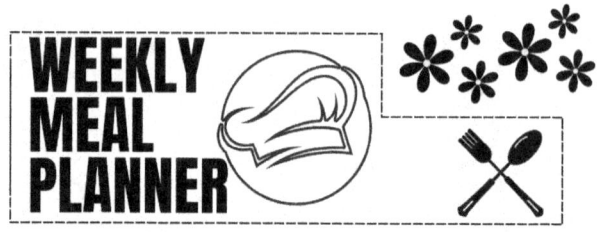

WEEKLY MEAL PLANNER

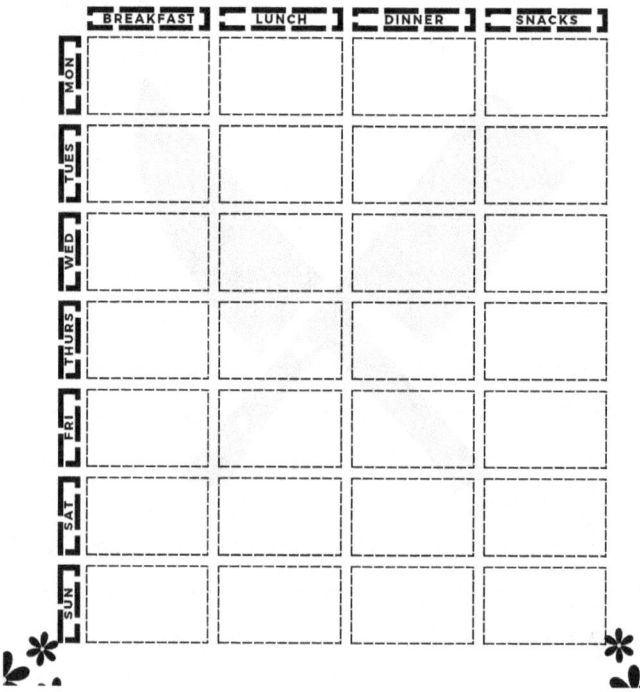

	BREAKFAST	LUNCH	DINNER	SNACKS
MON				
TUES				
WED				
THURS				
FRI				
SAT				
SUN				

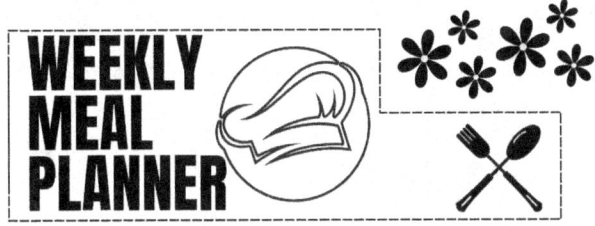

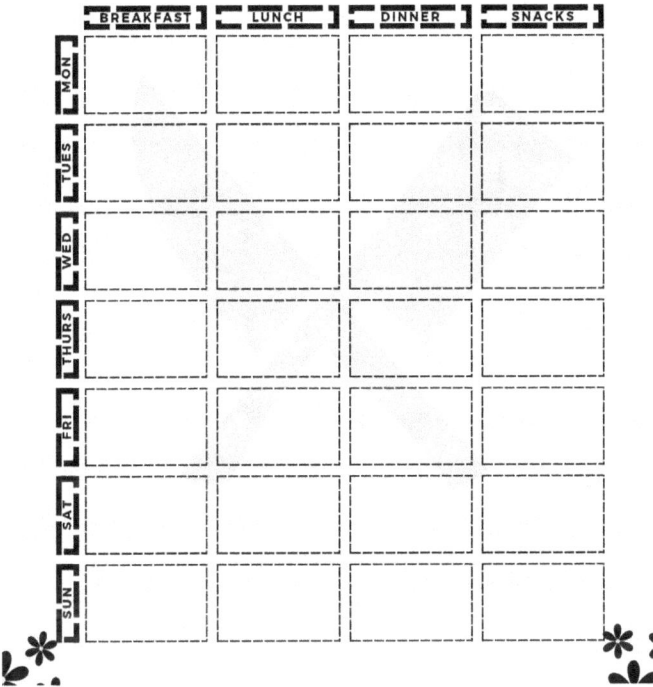

BREAKFAST	LUNCH	DINNER	SNACKS
MON			
TUES			
WED			
THURS			
FRI			
SAT			
SUN			

KIDNEY DIALYSIS DIET COOKBOOK FOR BEGINNERS

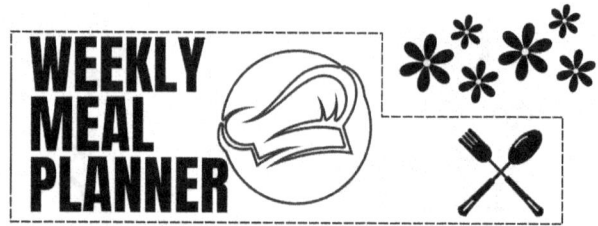

WEEKLY MEAL PLANNER

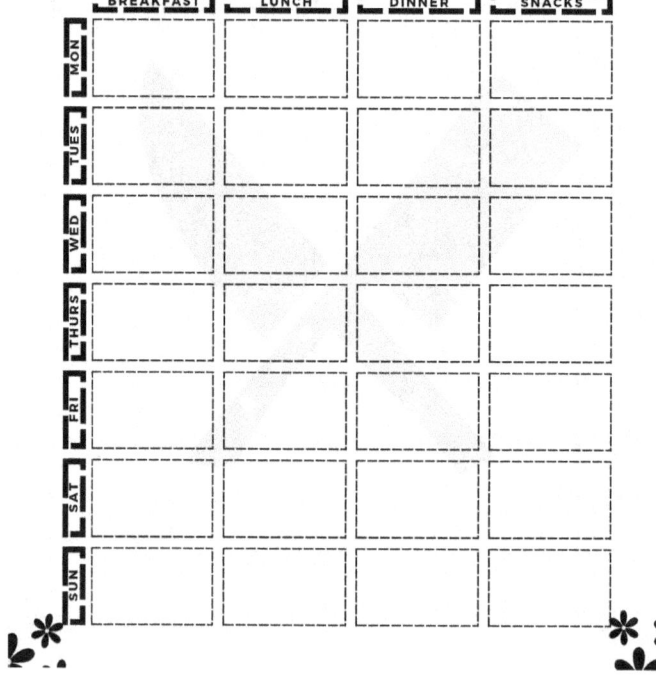

	BREAKFAST	LUNCH	DINNER	SNACKS
MON				
TUES				
WED				
THURS				
FRI				
SAT				
SUN				

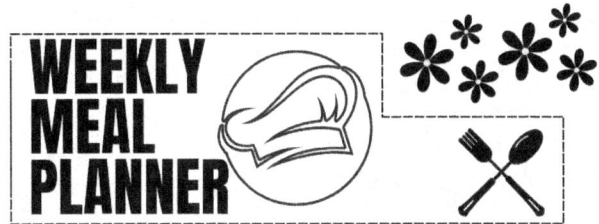

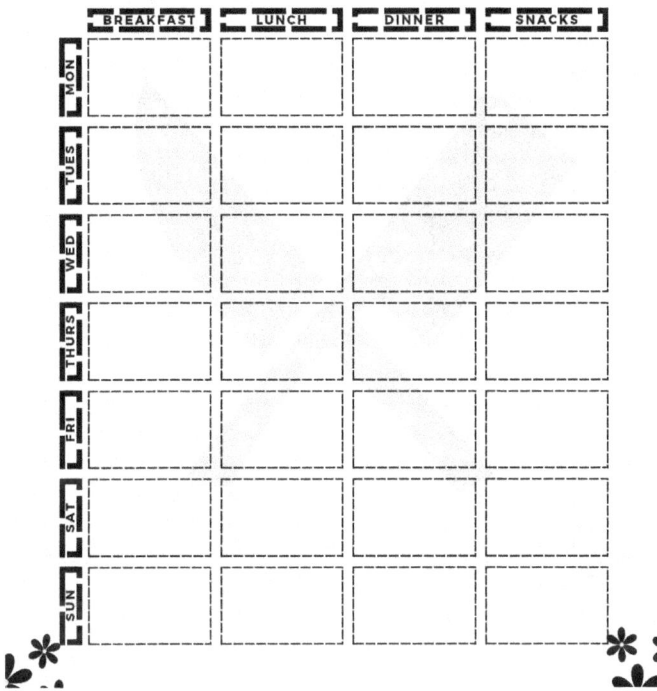

	BREAKFAST	LUNCH	DINNER	SNACKS
MON				
TUES				
WED				
THURS				
FRI				
SAT				
SUN				

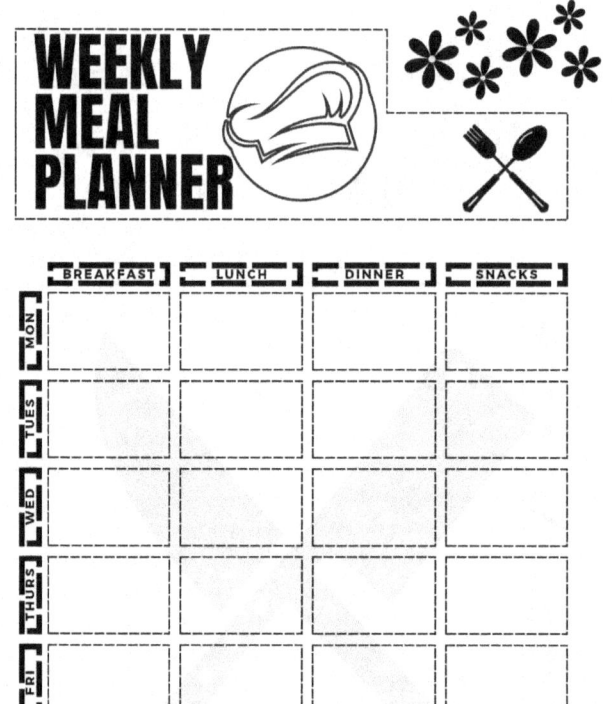

WEEKLY MEAL PLANNER

	BREAKFAST	LUNCH	DINNER	SNACKS
MON				
TUES				
WED				
THURS				
FRI				
SAT				
SUN				

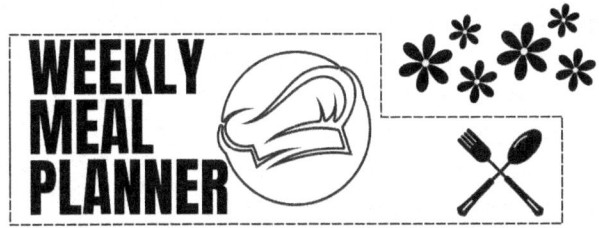

WEEKLY MEAL PLANNER

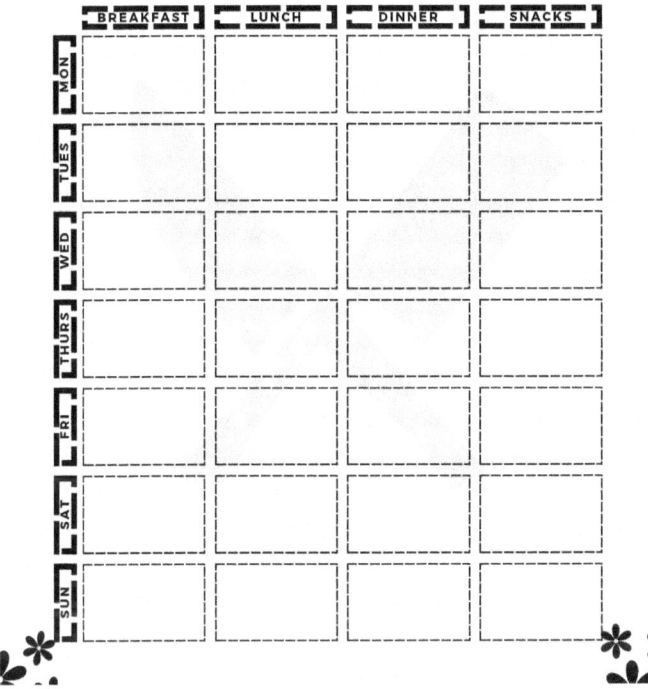

	BREAKFAST	LUNCH	DINNER	SNACKS
MON				
TUES				
WED				
THURS				
FRI				
SAT				
SUN				

www.ingramcontent.com/pod-product-compliance
Lightning Source LLC
Chambersburg PA
CBHW072207290526
45794CB00004B/1685